Let me explain:

Trying to lose weight to get healthy is putting the cart before the horse. Someone thinks, "Okay, then. I've got to get healthy. So, I will lose the weight. I'll drink protein shakes and only eat low-calorie frozen meals, soups, and salads with low-fat dressing. I'll do a 1,000 calorie a day diet. Then I can lose weight fast."

And here's where everything goes wrong, because when that doesn't work, they cut back to 800 calories. That is far too low a caloric intake for health and getting nutrients into your diet. The problem is that most people trying to lose weight start to cut calories and do it very unhealthily, substituting with things like:

- prepackaged soy-based protein powders
- super high-calorie, sugar-laden protein bars
- low-calorie nutrient-deficient high-carb meals (think frozen low-fat dinners)
- low-calorie but high-sugar foods, like many popular soups and flavored yogurts
- high-sugar/high-carb liquid diet shakes
- appetite suppressants, and
- stimulants that claim to block fat absorption, speed the metabolism, or even something new on the market I'm seeing—help make you more insulin sensitive (even if you're eating carbs!!)

But don't buy into it. Save your money for healthy choices.

Just ask any person who has yo-yo dieted most of their life—getting really thin and **then** gaining it back. They regain the weight over two to four years... but this time, they gain even MORE weight, reaching a new level of obesity they never thought they'd see on their frame. When you trim calories, not carbs—you end up with a body made of bones and fat. With a low-calorie high-carb intake, the body feeds off muscle.

This is why you see people burning off the legs and butt exercising and dieting without budging that huge middle. They're not tapping into fat burning. The dieters most obsessed with not eating FAT are the ones who are never actually LOSING FAT. You have to realize your weight is not THE problem but a symptom of something very unhealthy in your body. And this can occur despite all your blood tests coming out normal and your doctor saying, "Your tests are normal and you're healthy... JUST LOSE WEIGHT!"

Before we get into the #1 core problem, let's get deeper into what I mean by getting healthy. Let's start with the definition of the word FOOD:

***FOOD:** (n) that which is eaten to sustain life, provide energy, and promote the growth and repair of tissues; nourishment. [Old English foda, nourishment]*

Macmillan dictionary

We eat to:
1. Provide energy (fuel) and
2. Nourish the body (meaning to provide nutrients).

We can provide energy from sugar or fat as fuel. Sugar fuel is like running your body on diesel (dirty). Fat fuel is driving an expensive electric car—all powered up and running on clean, nontoxic fuel that powers your body with more energy than you've known in years... possibly decades.

The nutrients you need for health are vitamins, minerals, trace minerals, proteins, and healthy fats (fatty acids). Creating health starts with following the real definition of food!

BUT... We also need to **absorb** food (energy fuel and nutrients).

Actually **non-absorption** fuel and nutrients is the core issue. People are not absorbing nutrients at a cellular level anymore—because they are unhealthy. So their bodies are CRYING OUT for nutrients in the form of SUGAR and CARB cravings. That's just one part of the problem.

The key issue is this:

Most people use sugar as their cellular fuel. In fact, often, you may not even know how much sugar you ingest because it is hidden away in foods like tomato soup, cottage cheese, and low-fat/flavored yogurt, not to mention those tempting-looking boxes of cereal that look so nutrient-packed but are really packed with tons and tons of sugar.

See, the food we eat is digested and turns into glucose. This glucose then feeds the cells to provide energy. Vitamins and minerals provide helper factors—helping the body to make tissue, fortifying tissues like cells, and supporting the entire functioning of your body chemistry, from hormones, to metabolism, to the beating of your heart.

Amino acids (which make up proteins) supply fuel and the building blocks of hair, nails, skin, muscle, bone, etc., and fatty acids supply the surface of all your cells, nerves, and brain and act as the raw material for hormones.

The Core Problem

The body is constantly trying to survive and adapt to its environment and to new foods. It has a unique ability to convert from running on sugar fuel to running on fat fuel. This is ideal, and I'll get to this in a moment. In fact, once you know what that fat fuel feels like, you'll never go back to your old way of eating. You will love that feeling so much...

Back to how we're getting so unhealthy:
Our bodies do not have the ability to cope with or adapt to the overabundant and toxic amount of sugar we consume without creating LOTS of problems.

The core problem of the body today and the core problem causing this obesity—is **excess blood sugar**.

Why Your Body Will Do Anything to Fight Excess Sugar
The body will do nearly anything to maintain normal blood sugar and prevent excess. Normal blood sugar is a primary survival action and too much is a non-survival situation.

The main hormone that does MOST of this work to feed cells sugar AND prevent excess is...

INSULIN

What is insulin?
It is the body's chef that keeps everyone (all your cells) fed!
Insulin is a hormone (body communication) that is made by the pancreas, which is located under your left rib cage. Insulin's main function is to act as a key to allow cells to get energy fuel (glucose).

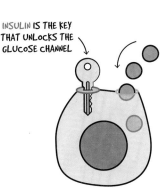

HOW DOES INSULIN WORK?

INSULIN

GLUCOSE

INSULIN IS THE KEY THAT UNLOCKS THE GLUCOSE CHANNEL

Insulin does four main things (and a lot more):

1. It **acts as a key** to open the door, allowing cells to get sugar fuel.
2. It **lowers excess sugar** in the blood after eating.
3. It **stores sugars** in the liver and muscles (glycogen).
4. And it **converts excess sugar** to fat and cholesterol.

In fact, insulin is THE main fat-making hormone.

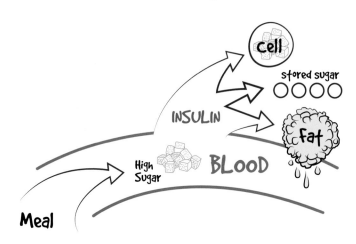

Insulin has some other vital functions, which we will get into later, but too much will make you fat AND prevent you from losing fat. Insulin mainly creates belly fat. And all fat burning is blocked in the presence of too much insulin.

*By the way, from here on out, I will use **glucose** and **sugar** interchangeably because they **are basically the same thing**.*

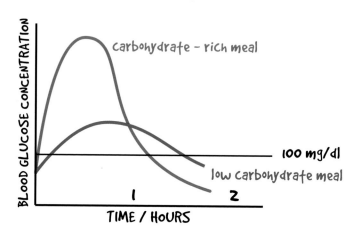

5

One trigger of insulin is a carbohydrate-rich meal. You eat, and the food turns into sugar, raising glucose in the blood, triggering insulin to whisk in to do its job to lower blood sugar, as seen in the next diagram.

What Does Normal Blood Sugar (100 mg/dl) Mean?

**When you get your blood sugar level tested,
normal should be between 90–100mg/dl.**

But what does that mean?

If your blood sugar is normal, it means that you have roughly one teaspoon of sugar (heaping) in all of your blood. An average person has about one and one-third gallons of blood in their body.

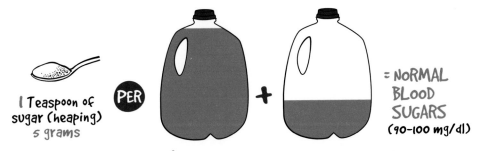

1 Teaspoon of
sugar (heaping)
5 grams

PER

+

= NORMAL
BLOOD
SUGARS
(90-100 mg/dl)

1 and 1/3 of a gallon of blood (avg. 165 lbs person)

As you can see, we don't need that much sugar in our blood, do we? In fact, that teaspoon of sugar can be made from non-carbohydrates, like dietary fat or protein. We really do not need to add any sugar to our bodies.

BUT… the average person in the US consumes **31 teaspoons of sugar each and every day!**

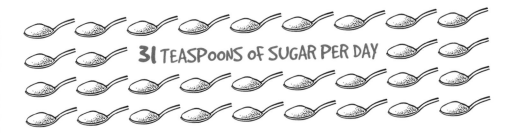

31 TEASPOONS OF SUGAR PER DAY

Just imagine how hard insulin has to work to remove this massively excessive amount of sugar from the blood!

Even more crazy is that the American Diabetes Association (ADA) recommends foods that equate to over 50 teaspoons of sugar per day. And the American Heart Association, the USDA Food Pyramid, and the Obesity Society all recommend a similar eating plan—high carbs. All that glucose. For someone with diabetes? Really?

FACT: Diabetes is too much sugar in the body.

What's wrong with this picture?

When you consume lots of sugar over time, your cells eventually start RESISTING and ignoring insulin. By doing this, insulin, the glucose key stops working which prevents excessive sugar in the cell. This is your body saying, "if you're going to keep eating sugar I will block it at the cell level."

Too Much Sugar Causes
Insulin Resistance

A sustained elevated blood sugar over time causes your cells to block or resist insulin. Your body considers sugar toxic and will protect you by stopping it from entering your cells. This is called insulin resistance. But since insulin is the KEY that controls cellular glucose, the cells can now become deprived of glucose.

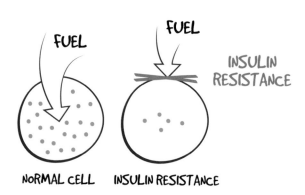

Insulin resistance is a prediabetic state. Since the cells need fuel but cannot get it, the pancreas has to compensate by making more insulin.

Insulin resistance makes your pancreas work too hard. In fact, insulin resistance forces the pancreas to make **5–7 times more insulin** that it should normally. So we have a situation where the body has way too much insulin in the blood—yet it's not working in the cells. The cells are resisting it. But the body keeps making more and more insulin. These hormones are on a constant feedback loop, sending and receiving messages of "sugar is high—release more insulin... must lower blood sugar for the body to stay alive."

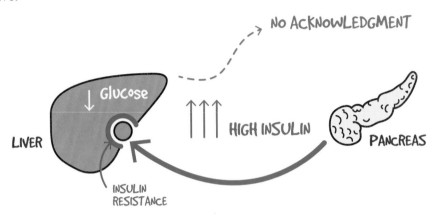

The problem is, the pancreas eventually becomes exhausted and makes less and less insulin—allowing the sugar in your blood to go higher and higher, requiring more and more medication, more glucose tests, more strips, and more needle sticks as well as highly impacting your quality of life. This is the story of diabetes.

All this happens gradually. It may not show up on blood tests until months or years later. In the meantime, however, insulin resistance symptoms may include…

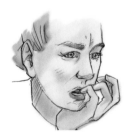
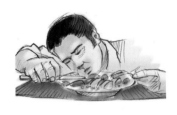
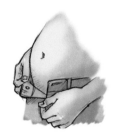

Anxiety   Tired After Meals   Belly Fat

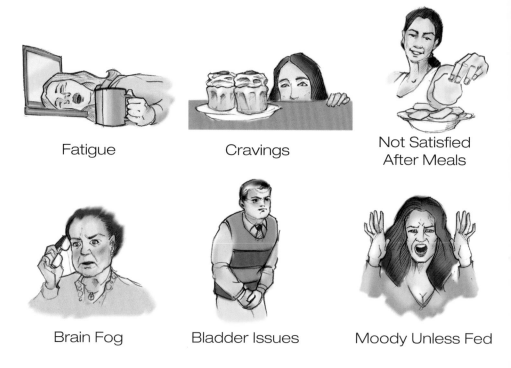

Fatigue

Cravings

Not Satisfied
After Meals

Brain Fog

Bladder Issues

Moody Unless Fed

These are also the symptoms of hypoglycemia (low blood sugar). Low blood sugar is also a prediabetic situation. The worst advice to give a hypoglycemic person is to have five to six meals a day. Yes, this will initially make the person feel better, but it continues the problem down the road.

Why?

Because eating triggers insulin! More on this in a moment. Insulin is the main fat-making hormone because it converts carbs into fat. This is especially true for belly fat and visceral fat (fat around the organs).

Fact: *If you see someone with belly fat, they have too much insulin!*

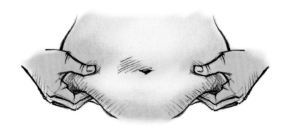

Okay, so now that you understand that, there is another VERY interesting function of insulin:

Cellular absorption of nutrients

Insulin is also needed to absorb potassium, magnesium, and amino acids. In fact, almost every nutrient is influenced by insulin. We need potassium for energy, balancing sodium in the body, and all kinds of other important things. We need amino acids for hair, nails, skin, joints and muscles. We need magnesium for a healthy heart... see where I am going?

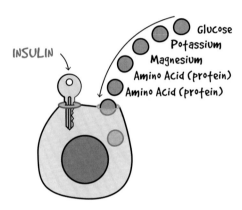

This means that when you have insulin resistance, you can become deficient in nutrients and protein, because they are not absorbed fully. Remember, health is created by providing nutrients and fuel and absorbing both.

But that's not all...
Insulin resistance can create deficiencies with:
1. Vitamin A
2. The B vitamins (especially B1 and B12)
3. Vitamin C
4. Vitamin D
5. Vitamin E
6. Vitamin K1 and K2
7. Calcium
8. Potassium
9. Magnesium
10. Omega-3 fatty acids

Getting all of these nutrients reduces insulin resistance, but insulin resistance can prevent cellular absorption of nutrients, a never ending cycle.

One of the terrible symptoms of diabetes is peripheral neuropathy, where the nerves in the feet and hands are destroyed, leading to burning pain and numbness. It could be pins and needles as well. This is a B1 and B12 deficiency.

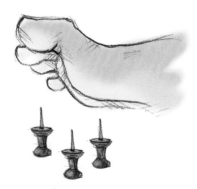

Insulin resistance causes vitamin C deficiency, in which the vascular system becomes a prime target of damage. If there is not enough vitamin C, you lose collagen to keep your arteries strong, triggering a cascade of events: LDL cholesterol, calcium, and white blood cells all start forming a bandage (plaque), which is known as a clogged artery.

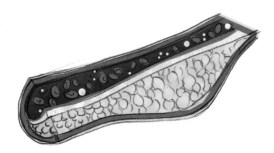

Vitamins A and D and even vitamins K1 and K2 all improve insulin resistance. Potassium, magnesium, and calcium also lessen the resistance of insulin working at the cellular level.

By the way, not to get off topic, but did you know that cancer and tumors can ***ONLY*** *live on sugar?*

Every single one of these problems listed below is connected to issues with INSULIN:

1. Type II diabetes
2. Heart disease
3. Stroke
4. High blood pressure
5. High cholesterol
6. Dementia and Alzheimer's
7. Fatty liver
8. And obesity (even though it's only a symptom)

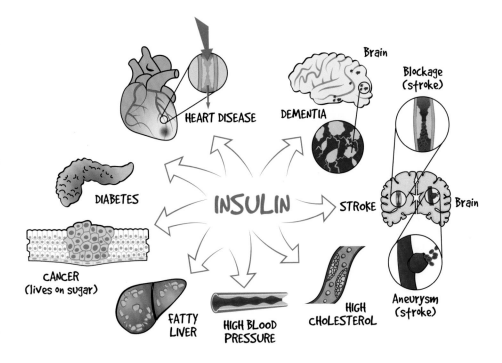

INSULIN RESISTANCE LEADS TO EXCESS INSULIN

High insulin is the underlying cause of the biggest health problems we experience.

The next question is…
HOW DO WE LOWER INSULIN?

#1 Eliminate the Sugar

This includes eliminating all sugar from the diet.

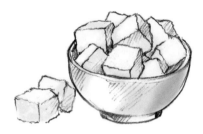

The key is bringing your dietary sugar down to zero! There are acceptable sweet alternatives. The three that I recommend that are easy to get are stevia, non-GMO erythritol, and non-GMO xylitol.

Avoid:

- Table sugar (cane and beet)
- Fructose
- Honey
- Brown sugar
- Agave nectar
- Dextrose
- Maltodextrin
- High-fructose corn syrup
- Maple syrup
- Rice syrup
- Juice
- Alcohol

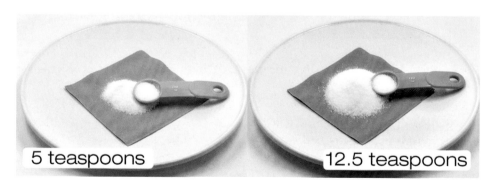

5 teaspoons   12.5 teaspoons

#2 Eliminate the Hidden Sugars

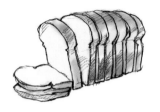 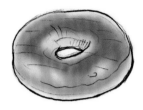 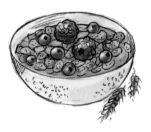

The four hidden carbohydrates that many people don't consider:

1. Grains
2. Starches
3. Fruits
4. Legumes (beans)

Grains to avoid include: breads, pasta, cereal (even oatmeal), crackers, biscuits, pancakes, and waffles. Even if something is gluten-free, it's still a grain. Gluten is the protein in grains.

You have to avoid ALL grains, including oats, wheat, barley, Ezekiel bread, sprouted bread and quinoa.

> *Exception: small amounts of This Crisp Rye Crispbread, a brand of rye crackers that only has four grams of sugar. This is net carbs, which is the total carbohydrate minus the fiber.*

Starches to avoid include: white and red potato, sweet potato, yams, white and brown rice, corn (even though it's a vegetable), and cornstarch.

Fruits to avoid include: apples, banana, pineapple, pear, dates, figs, grapes (and raisins), AND fruit juices (orange, grape, and apple juice—even tomato juice!).

> *Exception: small amounts (one-half to one cup) of berries per day.*

Legumes to avoid include: beans.

> *Exception: hummus.*

#3 Eliminate the Combination of Sugar or Refined Carbs with Protein

What's worse than consuming carbs? Combining sugar (or refined carbs) with protein can spike insulin by 200% more.

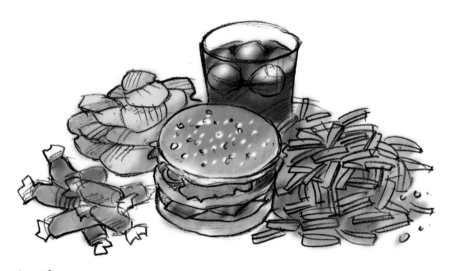

Avoid:

- Hamburger with bun
- Hot dog with bun
- Protein/bread combos in general
- Burger with fries
- Burger with ketchup (most condiments are packed with sugar, except for mustard!)
- Burger with soda
- Sweet and sour pork
- Breaded meats
- Beef jerky (unless it has no sugar)
- Deli meats (unless it has no sugar)
- Spaghetti and meatballs
- Lasagna
- Eggs and toast
- Sandwiches
- BBQ
- Chicken wings with sugary coating
- Cheese and crackers (except This Crisp Rye Crispbread)

#4 Eliminate MSG
(another hidden sugar)

Monosodium glutamate (MSG) is a flavor enhancer, meaning it makes food taste better than it usually does. It gives food a delicious savory flavoring. The way it works is to enlarge your taste buds to enhance the taste. It's in many, many foods at the grocery store and fast food restaurants, not to mention Chinese restaurants. You have to realize it can be listed under other names too: **modified cornstarch** and **modified starch**. So read your labels—even commercial cottage cheese has modified cornstarch.

MSG can spike insulin by 300%, even though it's not a carbohydrate.

#5 Eliminate Artificial Sweeteners

Avoid aspartame (Equal—it's also dangerous, and it's in many diet sodas) and saccharine (Sweet'N Low®). Even though these are sugar-free, they can spike insulin. Many people have been drinking diet soda for years without knowing the effects of these artificial sweeteners.

Sugar alcohols are much better: Non-GMO erythritol and xylitol are great. There are others, too. Stevia is the best, since it has a zero glycemic effect. You can even get soda-flavored xylitol that you can add to water to enjoy the taste of a soft drink without the insulin spike.

#6 Lean Proteins (low fat)

You may have already learned about this thing called the glycemic index (GI), but have you heard about the insulin index? This scale measures all the non-carbohydrate triggers of insulin. The big one is zero-fat protein, like in whey protein powder. This is interesting because we have been brainwashed into to eating low-fat everything. The fattier the meat, the lower the effect on insulin. So, when consuming protein, go for the higher-fat version—this includes cheese, dairy, meats, fattier fish, etc. It would also be better to leave the skin on the chicken if possible.

#7 Excessive Proteins

Another trigger of insulin is large quantities of protein. This was one of the issues with the Atkins diet. The optimum amount of protein per meal should be three to six ounces. Protein is needed for repairing and providing the raw material for muscle, tendons, joint cartilage, and even bone. Protein can also be used for fuel; however, too much triggers insulin and can be converted to sugar and then to fat.

A common question people have is "Should I not be consuming lots of protein to build my muscles?" The liver can only handle so much, and keeping your protein to a moderate amount is all you need.

#8 Eating Too Frequently

Did you realize that eating in general triggers insulin? It is not a good idea to eat five to six small meals per day. This spikes insulin big-time and prevents you from correcting insulin resistance. The solution to this is intermittent fasting (IF); more on this later.

The Solution

There are two strategies I recommend to lose weight and reverse insulin resistance:

- Healthy Ketosis and
- Intermittent Fasting

Healthy Ketosis

This is a healthy state in which the body is using ketones as its primary fuel. Ketones are the by-product of fat and a much cleaner fuel. Ketones are the preferred fuel of the body and brain. Running on glucose is inefficient for the body and unhealthy in numerous ways—it is also a recent development for humankind.

When people try to lose weight, they usually lose some initial water weight and plateau after two weeks. They rarely tap into fat fuel.

Healthy ketosis emphasizes getting your required nutrients. In the most advanced form of diabetes (type I), a condition called *ketoacidosis* exists. This is completely different from ketosis. Ketoacidosis is a disease state where there is no more insulin and acids build up to high levels that are dangerous for health. But with ketosis, the pH in the body never even gets close to the high levels seen with ketoacidosis.

Ketosis is the state of running your body on FAT!

The benefits are immense... and go way beyond weight loss.

By running on fat fuel with ketosis, you'll experience rewards like:

- No more cravings
- Less hunger between meals
- Better memory
- Cardiovascular protection
- Normal blood sugar
- Improved mood
- Improved cholesterol
- Way more energy
- Amazing skin
- Much less inflammation
- Improved sleep

To get into a state of ketosis so you can run on fat instead of glucose—and finally burn your own fat stores for fuel—you will have to start adapting your body to fat burning! You have to switch the body's preferred fuel source. For some people, this can take as long as six weeks, while for others, it only takes one to two weeks.

But you want to finally get that fat off the body, yes? This is the way to do it! Finally, you'll lose weight, while getting healthy and preserving lean muscle, so you can burn more calories every day—unlike the muscle you lose by running on sugar and NEVER tapping into fat burning.

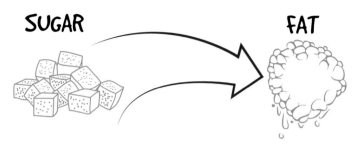

SUGAR

FAT

How Does Ketosis Work?

The key to switching your body to fat burning is to lower your carb intake to 20–50 grams per day. People who have a very slow metabolism might have to go even lower and keep the carb intake around 20 grams or less.

By the way, there is no such thing as an "essential carbohydrate." Our bodies can do quite well without carbohydrates. There are different types of carbohydrates: vegetables, fruits, berries, starches (potato and rice), grains, and legumes. Then you have the really bad guys—refined carbohydrates like table sugar, wheat flour, and high-fructose corn syrup.

With ketosis, we want to stick to vegetables and very small amounts of berries only. Vegetables give us our vitamins and minerals and turn into sugar **very slowly**. Berries turn into sugar much more slowly than fruit.

Consuming fruit and fruit juices is the worst. And did you know that an apple contains a whopping 19 grams of sugar?

Intermittent Fasting

Intermittent fasting (IF) is not a diet. It is limiting the frequency of meals, allowing you to rely on fat burning for all the time between eating your meals and while you're sleeping at night.

This is important because one of the primary triggers of insulin is EATING—eating anything. So eating five to six times a day—and let's not forget, snacking will spike insulin. Frequent eating through the day causes chronic sustained higher levels of insulin, and this leads to insulin resistance.

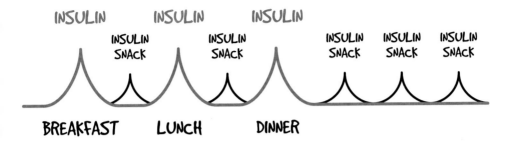

Eating less often with no snacks to spike insulin in between meals is **the most powerful way** to correct insulin resistance.

To do this, first start with three meals per day—NO snacks—absolutely nothing between meals but water, black coffee, and other non-caloric, non–insulin spiking drinks. (Too much coffee, however, will also spike insulin.)

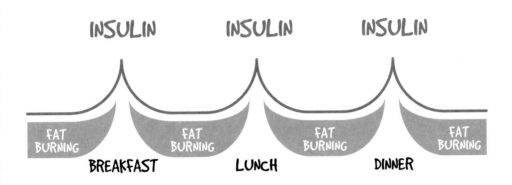

Keeping insulin at normal between meals and during sleep allows the pancreas to rest and recover. But some people have a hard to time going from one meal to the next because they get blood sugar crashes and severe hunger.

The solution to this is to consume more fat at the meal. Fat not only satisfies you the most but triggers insulin the least. Consuming lean protein and low-fat meals keeps you hungry, so the answer is more fat.

The goal over time is to GRADUALLY transition from three meals per day to a shortened daily eating window by eating only two meals a day.

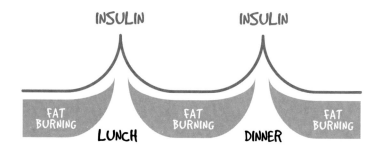

This is not about lowering your calorie intake; it's about eating less often. Your new goal should be to reduce the frequency of meals you eat and avoid spiking insulin.

Again, **low-calorie diets do not work** because they keep you hungry and craving—even worse, they deprive you of nutrients, eventually slowing your metabolism. If you're transitioning from three to two meals, make sure your two meals contain the same calories as the three meals.

Think about it—you are training your body to run on your own body fat as its fuel source between meals.

The secret is to do it gradually. The main reason for going slowly is that your body needs time to build up the cellular machinery and enzymes to burn fat or shall I say ketones. Ketones are the byproduct of fat burning.

Start with three meals a day, no snacks. And then gradually postpone breakfast further and further until you can skip it all together. For example, in the diagram below, your first meal could be at 10:00am and your last meal at 6:00 pm, giving you an eight-hour eating window.

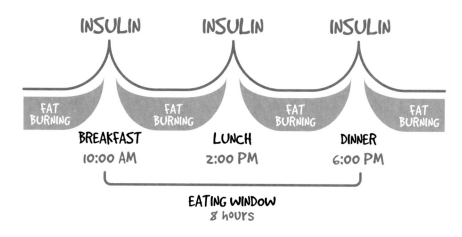

As you adapt, which is called *keto-adaptation* (and can take two to four weeks), it will be easier to go longer before your first meal. Continue to shorten your eating window as gradually as you can, as seen in the diagram below with a four-hour eating window as seen below. There are many different combinations. My wife will wait until 3:00 pm before her first meal, but will eat a later dinner around 7:00-8:00 pm. This could take some time to achieve but is very effective for weight loss.

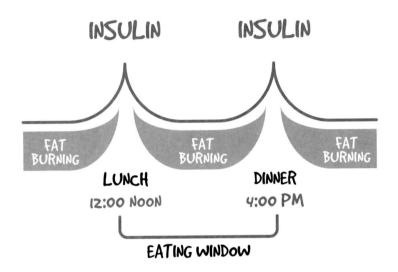

It is okay to be a *little* hungry as long as it does not impair your cognitive function or cause headaches or weakness.

In other words, allow your body to adjust to running on fat. For some true sugar junkies, this can take a few months. Your cells will eventually adjust, you'll enter full fat-burning mode, and then it gets really, really easy to resist snacking because you have no cravings and not really hungry anymore. And when you see the weight just melting off, this will motivate you to stick to your new way of eating.

I found that you'll need more fat with meals at first but as you burn more of your own fat, you'll need less. Some people decide to even do one meal per day especially if the thyroid is very slow. But with one meal a day, just make sure the meal is a robust one, containing all the needed nutrients to fortify your body with vitamins, minerals, amino acids, those important fatty acids, trace minerals—all of it. (This can be aided with green drink powders and high-quality electrolyte supplements that will help you get your daily requirements for potassium.

Intermittent Fasting is a very healthy thing to do because it increases the anti-aging and muscle-preserving growth hormone by up to 2000%.

It also helps regrow brain cells improving cognitive function.

Getting All Your Nutrients

This is the third piece of the puzzle. Part of getting healthy is getting the required nutrients. Fixing insulin resistance allows you to absorb your nutrients even better, but you still need to get all the nutrients you need from the food you eat.

If you research ketogenic diets or even IF, you'll notice that there is not an emphasis on fulfilling nutrient requirements. This is where a lot of proponents of keto and IF go wrong—they should emphasize the nutrient density aspect because this is what ultimately gets your body and your metabolism healthy.

Generally speaking, most of the vitamins and minerals you will need come from vegetables. B vitamins are present in whole wheat, but these grains turn into sugar too fast so we will get our B vitamins from other foods. Nutritional yeast is high in B-vitamins.

Certain vitamins in vegetables—especially the fat-soluble vitamins like vitamin A—only come in a pre-vitamin form. This means when you eat pre–vitamin A rich foods, like carrots or spinach, the pre-vitamin form has to be converted into the active form of vitamin A, and you're only going to get roughly 4% of the active form of vitamin A. This is why it's recommended to consume high quality animal sources including grass fed meats and dairy.

By the way, the best sources of the active form of vitamin A are egg yolk, cod liver oil, fatty fish, butter, grass-fed liver, and grass-fed dairy. Vitamin D can come from the sun, cod liver oil, egg yolk, and grass-fed dairy.

Vitamin K2, another fat-soluble vitamin, is crucial to keep calcium out of the soft tissues and in your bones. Vitamin K2 comes from grass-fed dairy, cheese, egg yolk, and liver.

Potassium is that mineral you need the most. It's also the hardest to get in the diet. You have to really focus on it.

Our bodies need 4,700 mg of potassium every single day. Bananas only have 300 mg of potassium, plus all that sugar. You would have to consume more than 15 bananas a day just to meet the potassium requirements. But that won't work to help you burn fat, because of all that sugar you'd be eating.

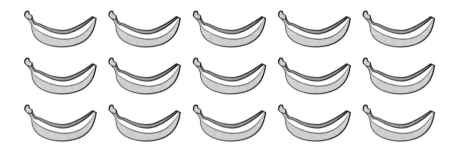

Avocados and beet tops (beet greens) have lots of potassium and all kinds of other vitamins and minerals that are good for you.

I recommend getting your potassium from leafy greens, but you're going to have to consume larger salads. I recommend consuming seven to ten cups of salad per day. This will not only provide you with a good amount of potassium but most of the rest of the required nutrients as well.

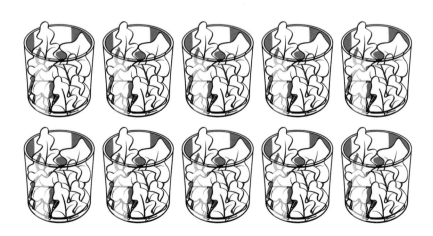

If you go shopping for salad, realize that one cup equals one ounce. Bags of salad are often five ounces (five cups) and plastic containers are also five ounces, to give you a reference.

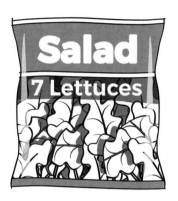
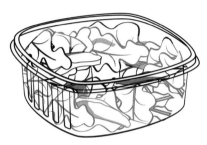

Consuming large salads with spring mix, spinach, arugula or even cabbage will start to give you the nutrients that help undo insulin resistance. There are numerous studies that demonstrate that various nutrients (Vitamin A, B, C, D, K, potassium, magnesium, and chromium) improve insulin resistance. Adding in intermittent fasting will also help insulin dysfunction, which is the icing on the cake…sorry, I couldn't withhold that one.

Below are some examples of amounts of salad.

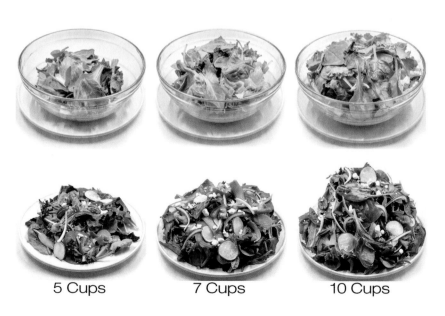

5 Cups   7 Cups   10 Cups

Keto-Adaptation

Your body is going to have to switch fuel sources and will need new cellular process to accomplish this. By following this plan, your cells will change over and adapt; however, it takes some time, usually one to four weeks. It all depends on how serious your insulin resistance is.

During this adjustment phase, you might experience some of the following symptoms:

1. Keto flu (feeling rundown)
2. Fatigue
3. Irritability
4. Muscle cramps
5. Kidney stones
6. Sleep problems
7. Constipation
8. Keto rash

Generally speaking, to help reduce these symptoms, there are two main types of nutrients you need: B vitamins and electrolytes!

Electrolytes are minerals like potassium, calcium, magnesium, sodium and chlorides.

For B vitamins, I recommend nutritional yeast, which is packed with virtually all the B vitamins you need every day but make sure it's unfortified. When they fortify nutritional yeast, they use synthetic vitamins.

It is very difficult to pinpoint exactly which mineral or vitamin is needed for a specific symptom you may experience when you start to adapt. That's why the one product I highly recommend is my electrolyte powder.

It contains 1000 mg of potassium per serving, not to mention all other minerals as well as trace minerals but without the maltodextrin (or sugar) that normally comes with most electrolyte powders.

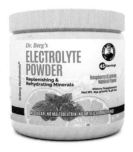

Putting It All Together

We are going to combine nutrient-dense foods, ketosis, and IF to achieve maximum weight loss and health. Let's start with what to eat and give you plenty of examples, okay?

What to Eat

Most people need to consume between 1500–2100 total calories per day, depending on the size of the body. To make this simple, all the meal examples I give and macro ratios (protein, carbs fats) are based on 1800 calories per day. Of course, this is just for an average adult. You'll want to adjust caloric intake based on your body size and activity level, however I would you prefer not to count your calories. Since the purpose of food is to get nutrients, calories may or may not give you nutrients. But I know someone will ask about how many calories they need, so here you go!

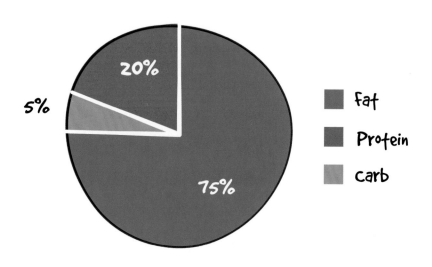

Protein Amounts

On average, you will be consuming three to six ounces of protein at each meal. What does this look like? See below!

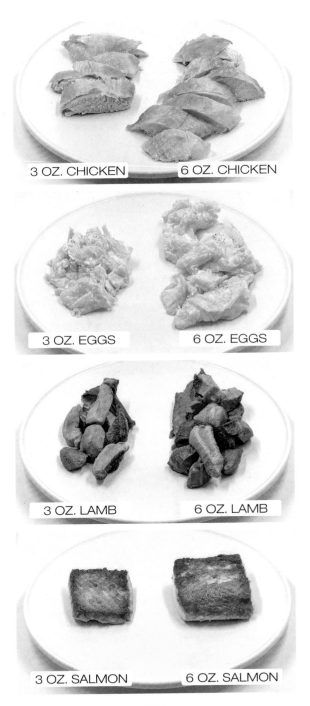

3 OZ. CHICKEN — 6 OZ. CHICKEN

3 OZ. EGGS — 6 OZ. EGGS

3 OZ. LAMB — 6 OZ. LAMB

3 OZ. SALMON — 6 OZ. SALMON

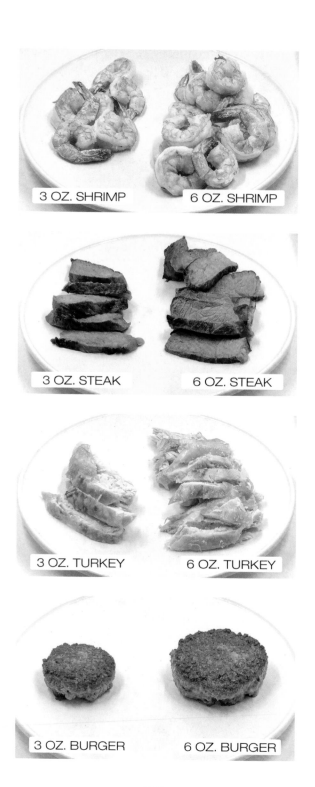

If you are doing three meals a day, here is an example of how much TOTAL protein you could eat in one day.

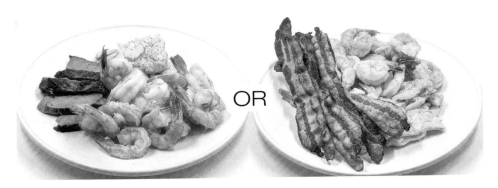

Carbohydrate Amounts

You want to keep your carbohydrate amounts between 20 and 50 grams per day. Many people use 30 grams to keep it simple, but the lower the carbohydrates, the greater the fat burning. When we deal with vegetables, we have the total carbohydrate amounts and the fiber. If you deduct the fiber from the total carbohydrates, you get net carbohydrates. You want to use net carbs for your calculations, not total carbs.

Because vegetables are so high in fiber, the net carbs they yield are very low. I do not recommend you limit or even factor in your vegetable carbohydrates when calculating total carbohydrates. In fact, go for larger amounts of vegetables instead, seven to ten cups per day. The exception is higher-sugar vegetables: carrots, beets, tomatoes, corn (avoid if GMO), peas, onions, and sweet peppers.

Also, remember that even foods that don't seem like it do have carbs, like nuts, seeds, and hummus, actually contain carbs. Berries have less sugar than other fruits. That's why are allowable on the keto program.

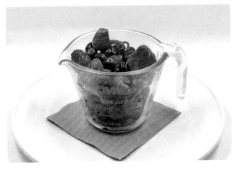

Fat Amounts

When you calculate 75 percent of your total calories per day, it may initially seem like a lot. However, because fat has almost double the calories than proteins and carbs, it's not that much. Here are a few examples of what total daily fat for the day looks like.

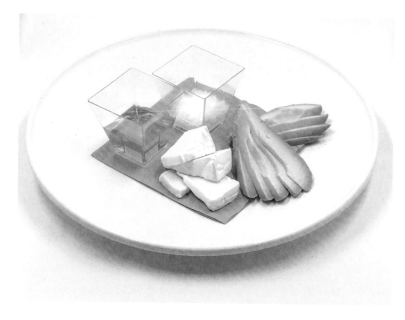

or

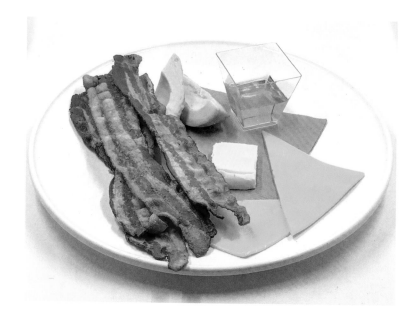

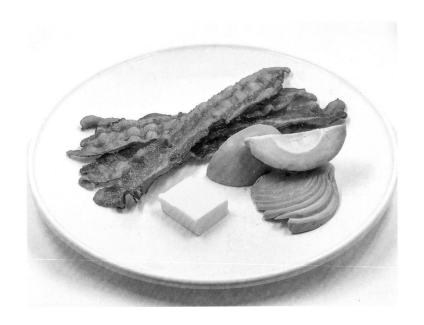

or

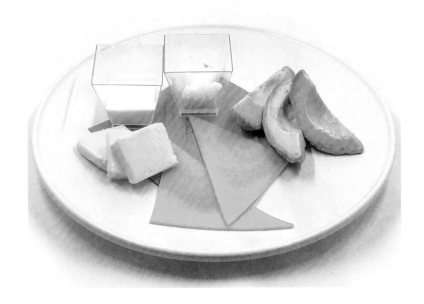

Meal Examples

The meal above is a good example of the percentages of macros you need. The only thing I would add to this meal is more veggies or salad.

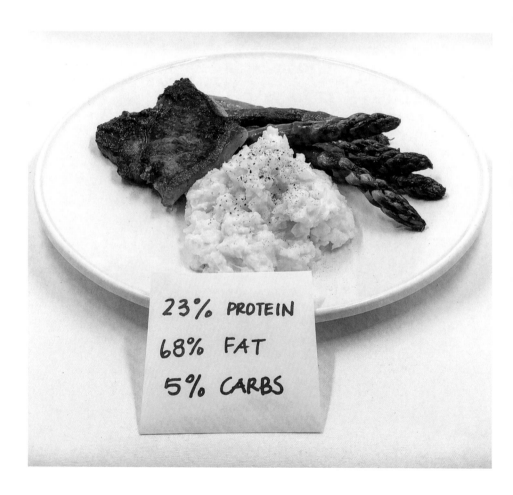

23% PROTEIN
68% FAT
5% CARBS

3-Meal Examples

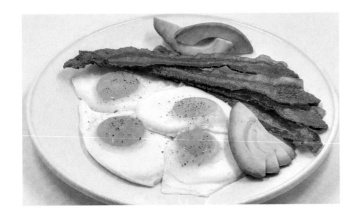

Breakfast

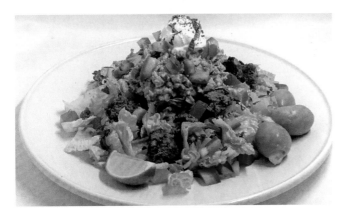

Lunch

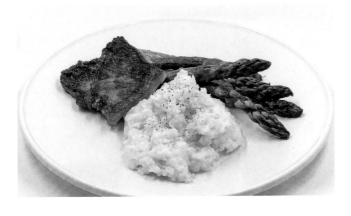

Dinner

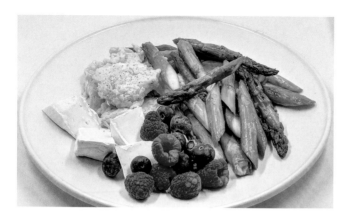

Breakfast

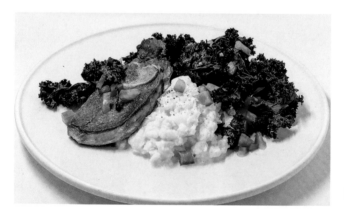

Lunch

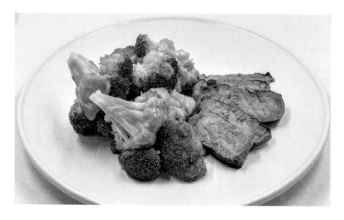

Dinner

35

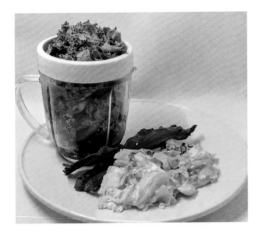

Breakfast

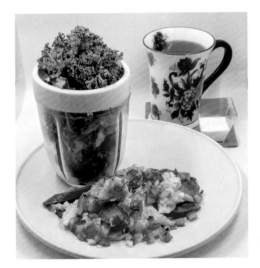

Lunch

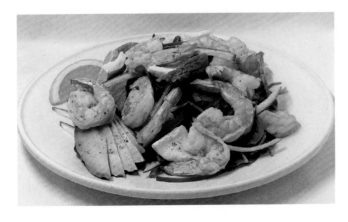

Dinner

36

2-Meal Examples

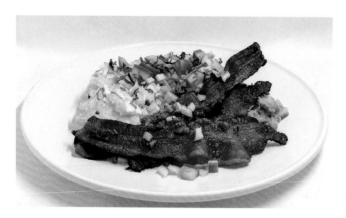

First Meal

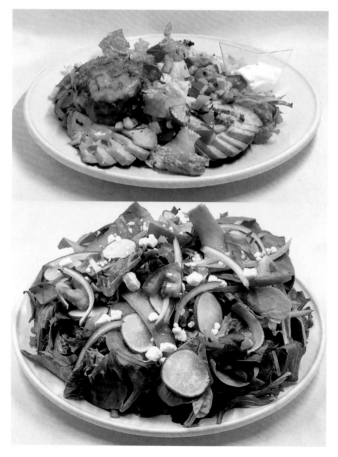

Second Meal

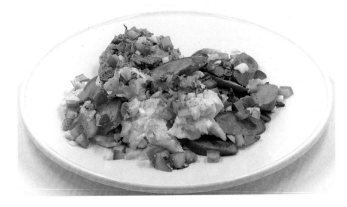

First Meal

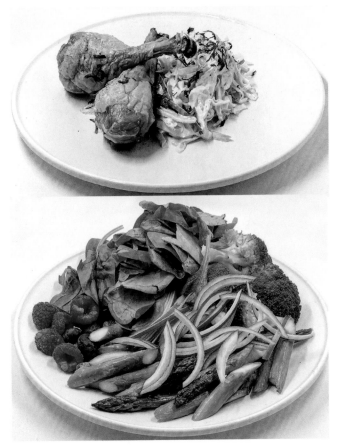

Second Meal

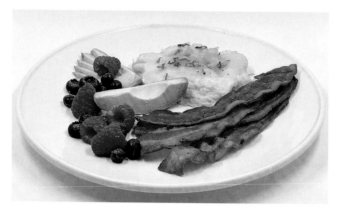

First Meal

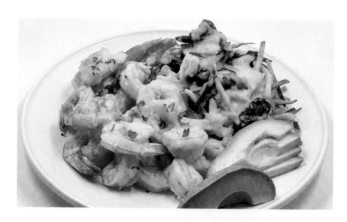

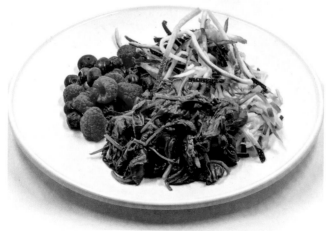

Second Meal

39

Frequently Asked Questions on Ketosis and Intermittent Fasting

What is a ketone?

A ketone is a byproduct of fat being burned. It is basically an alternative source of energy (fuel) from glucose. Ketones are the preferred fuel for the body and more efficient for the brain and the heart.

How long before I start losing weight?

A lot of times, people want this to start happening right now. Your body has been running on glucose for your entire life, though. Your cells have to build new enzymes—a whole new cellular machine, to break down fat as a new source of fuel. It may happen in a month, but more likely, it will take at least six weeks. But once you do get there—you won't have sugar cravings anymore. You'll have better blood sugar. Your memory will be sharper and you'll urinate less at night and sleep better because your blood sugar won't be plummeting during the night after sugar spikes.

Okay, I "fell off the wagon" and cheated.
How long will it take me to get back into ketosis now?

It can take 48–72 hours if you're lucky, but it could be up to a week. Now, if you're in your twenties and pretty healthy, you'll bounce right back in a day. When you're older and working on repairing a broken metabolism, it will take longer.

I started the keto diet about a week ago. Now I'm tired constantly. What do I do?

As your body adjusts to fat burning, you will need more B vitamins. The nutrient you need a lot of to keep the fatigue away and help your adrenals and metabolism is B5. A sodium deficiency could also produce fatigue and weakness.

How can I avoid (or get over) the keto flu?

The symptoms of keto flu are headaches, body aches, cravings, brain fog, and fatigue. Just think about what you're trying to do. You're converting your ENTIRE cellular machinery to fat burning. What you need to do to avoid or heal the keto flu is get more electrolytes and B vitamins.

These are the cofactors that help in developing the machinery to burn fat effectively without draining your body. For the B vitamins, try nutritional yeast. However, nutritional yeast does not have B5—so you may have to take a B5 supplement. I recommend my electrolyte powder.

It has 1,000 mgs of potassium and will help you get to 4,700 mgs you need to create this machinery to burn fat faster and get into ketosis!

Will too much protein throw me out of ketosis?

Yes, especially too much lean protein—like turkey and chicken and even lean fish. Egg white without the yolk is lean protein and will trigger insulin more than the whole egg. Normally three to six ounces of protein is sufficient, and 10+ ounces is going to kick you out of ketosis.

I heard that on a ketosis diet you eat more fat—isn't that unhealthy?

A lot of conflicting information has been circulated about the consumption of fat. People are sometimes concerned that adding fat to their diet will cause them to gain weight. This is not necessarily the case. Fat is a neutral food when it comes to insulin. It is also satisfying. Fat allows you to feel full for longer to help with IF.

Are condiments bad for ketosis?

Actually, YES. Ketchup, BBQ sauce, and Asian sauces like duck sauce and sweet and sour sauce are LOADED with sugar, and eating sugar with protein greatly spikes INSULIN—exactly what you don't want to do. Mustard is okay. Mayonnaise is okay if not made with soy. Start looking at sugar grams on EVERYTHING, especially your salad dressings.

Does ketosis worsen adrenal health?

No. Ketosis allows your adrenal glands to function more stably.
It works like this:

The adrenal glands make cortisol, which is triggered by stress. Cortisol increases insulin, which will kick you out of ketosis. When you decrease insulin (as with ketosis), you lower stress and lower cortisol. Therefore, the adrenal glands don't have to work so hard and will function more healthily.

I love hummus. Will that throw me out of ketosis?

No—hummus is great for ketosis. The six basic ingredients of hummus are all very good for you. Just be sure to avoid hummus with preservatives and/or soybean oil. Look for hummus that contains only chickpeas, tahini, olive oil, garlic, lemon, and sea salt.
Also, you'll want to eat your hummus with vegetables, not chips or pita bread.

Does ketosis cause hypothyroidism?

The short answer is no. A low-carbohydrate diet is not the thing that causes a slow thyroid. A low-calorie diet, however, can cause hypothyroidism. Sometimes, people on a ketosis diet will find that they're just not that hungry. So if you're going to do a ketosis diet, you need to make sure you provide your body with enough nutrients.

Will vegetables slow ketosis?

I get asked this question a lot. Generally speaking, the answer is no. As long as you avoid vegetables like corn, beets, and carrots, which are high in starch and sugar (especially carrot JUICE, which is packed with sugar), you don't have to worry about the vegetable family.

In fact, you want to eat lots of green leafy vegetables, cruciferous vegetables and Brussel sprouts. Create big kale salads with bacon bits and a full-fat dressing. Or make a big beet greens sautéed in coconut oil with some bacon, garlic, and onion stirred in. These will be dishes PACKED with potassium, which will quiet food cravings much like fat does. Often, food cravings are nothing more than your body crying out for NUTRIENTS and MINERALS you're not giving it.

Should I count total carbs or net carbs?

Count the net carbs, which is total carbs minus fiber.

Is it possible to eat too much fat?

Yes. If you look up the ketosis diet online, they say to consume 85% of calories from fat. If you consume 2500 calories from fat, you are consuming 220 grams of fat per day. I believe this is excessive and could prevent fat burning because then you'd be running on the fat you're consuming rather than your fat stores. In the beginning you'll need more fat to go from one meal to the next; however, as you fully adapt, you'll need less because you'll run on your own body's fat.

How much fat should I eat at each meal?

If you're really battling a high appetite/high craving day or week, you might want to add more fat, especially at breakfast to trim your appetite throughout the day and enable you to go longer without cravings and hunger.

Ketosis in general suppresses your appetite, so your hunger will be greatly reduced. You're going to be able to go many hours without eating. Let the hunger dictate how much fat you eat. If you're not hungry, cut down on the fat a little bit.

What about keto bombs? What are these?

Keto bombs are a fat cookie that ketogenic dieters love because they're healthy, delicious cheat foods that are virtually devoid of carbs.

I have a lot of videos on how to make keto bombs, but you have to have them with a meal, not as a snack. The goals would be to stick to one a day. Go to my YouTube channel under playlists and recipes.

What are the seven reasons ketosis is superior for weight loss and health?

You're running your body on ketones, not glucose, and...

1. Ketones are a superior fuel.
2. Ketosis produces the most weight loss of any diet I know of, targeting the belly in particular.
3. Ketosis improves your memory and cognitive function. Awesome for kids that have epilepsy. Great for Alzheimer's or Parkinson's.
4. Ketosis improves mood. When running on sugar, you get highs and lows; you're irritable and grouchy all the time.
5. Ketosis eradicates cravings and hunger. It's crazy to try to diet when you're hungry and have cravings. When you're running on ketones, you don't have that fluctuation of blood sugar.
6. Ketosis improves metabolism, can repair a set point that is stuck at a certain weight, and will allow you to bust through that plateau.
7. Ketosis improves insulin dysfunction.

So ketosis is very powerful for health and can even help prevent or reverse insulin resistance, prediabetes, high blood pressure, Polycystic Ovarian Syndrome (PCOS), and kidney stones.

I am losing NO weight. Why?

You may be losing fat and gaining muscle, which is a bit heavier thus no actual weight loss. I would use midsection weight rather than weight as your indicator of whether it's working.

I've heard ketosis can cause kidney stones. Is there anything we can do to prevent this from happening?

People on a ketosis diet may be at higher risk for kidney stones, but these are easily preventable. Here's how it can happen:

With a ketosis diet, you tend to eliminate more calcium than usual. Additionally, foods such as cruciferous vegetables, spinach, iced tea, or chocolate all have a high amount of oxalates. Oxalates are naturally occurring substances found in a wide variety of foods; they play a supportive role in the metabolism of many plants and animals, including humans. Oxalates combined with calcium can cause kidney stones.

Lemon juice contains citrates (the substance that gives citrus fruits their sour taste). When you're low on citrates, you're at risk for kidney stones. Add the lemon juice to your kale shake or drink it in water. Try to consume at least one lemon per day (lemon juice or the fruit of the lemon).

I also recommend taking my electrolyte mix, as it contains minerals in their citric form as in potassium citrate, helping to bind the oxalate stones and neutralize uric acid stones.

I've heard ketogenic diets can get rid of migraines. Is this true?

Yes. Eliminating insulin spikes has been shown to greatly reduce migraines. Adding IF, in fact, speeds this process even more. Your brain will be less stressed using ketones as fuel.

What are the biggest mistakes people make when doing ketosis?

Eating too much or too little fat! If you don't eat enough fat, you won't be successful because a) too little fat is unhealthy and b) fat helps control the appetite. So this is the wild variable that needs to be figured out as you experiment with your body.

Can you be in ketosis and not show it on your urine test?

There are three kinds of ketones, and the urine only tests for acetoacetate. As you switch to more efficient fat-burning process, you convert that acetoacetate to beta-hydroxybutyrate. So, yes, you can actually show negative or zero ketones. Look at other factors. Are you losing weight? Are you feeling good? If you're doing 20 grams net carbs a day or less, you're going to be in ketosis, no matter what.

What about fruit on a ketogenic diet? Can I do it?

In short, no. Even apples have too many carbs. Pineapples will create massive insulin spikes. Never consume fruit juices. The fiber is bound to the phytonutrients and the juice is cooked, removing many nutrients. You're basically just drinking concentrated fructose. You can get away with one-half to one cup of berries a day.

What about nuts and seeds on keto?

Nuts and seeds are fine. Macadamias and pecans are great fatty nuts. (But walnuts and macadamias can go rancid. Be careful.) Cashews are higher in carbohydrates, so avoid them. For nut butters, look on the label. You want sea salt and peanuts or almonds only. Make sure there's no added food starch or MSG. MSG really spikes INSULIN.

Two to three ounces of nuts in a given meal should be fine – but less if you have a gallbladder issue. Seeds are even better than nuts, nutrition wise. Chia seeds, flax seeds, sunflower seeds—they're high in healthy nutrients, high in fat, low in carbs—they're good for you. You can put them on salads, make a trail mix, all kinds of neat stuff you can do!

Is gluten-free healthy on a keto diet?

It's true, gluten is harmful to the gut. But just because a food doesn't have gluten, doesn't mean it's safe; you're still dealing with the wheat, which turns into sugar quickly. Quinoa, buckwheat, sorghum, millet—all these have similar effects as wheat, so avoid them.

What other things will kick me out of ketosis?

1. Stress elevates insulin. Calming strategies work! Stress activates cortisol, which can keep you from weight loss as well.

2. Caffeine elevates stress in the body—again.
Also, adrenaline spikes insulin.

3. Too much bone broth. Too much protein in general is a risk.
It's a small risk, though.

4. Bloating from kale and other vegetables that you have
a hard time digesting.

Is coffee okay on the ketogenic diet?

Sure, if you're having about one 8 ounce cup per day, not 15 cups. The problem with coffee is that it is the third most sprayed crop in the world AND it depletes the adrenals. If you're going to do coffee, make sure it's organic, that the creamer is organic, and that you use XYLITOL—which is GMO-free and tastes just like sugar.

Is decaf coffee all right?

Be careful with decaf—Companies use the chemical methyl chloride to remove caffeine. You want to buy coffee utilizing CO_2 and the Water Process, pioneered by SWISS WATER®

Can I eat oatmeal on a ketogenic diet or will it bump me out of fat burning?

Steel-cut oats (unrefined) are better than instant oats on the glycemic index scale. However, it's still too high for keto, and will slow you down. Instant oatmeal is around 83 on the GI. It will turn into a LOT of sugar. If

you're trying to lose weight, oatmeal WILL slow you down, so no.

Is stevia okay on a ketogenic diet?

Yes, pure stevia is fine. Stevia with maltodextrin is not good, so read the labels.

Will diet soda throw me out of ketosis?

The artificial sweeteners in soda are not only bad for you but also spike insulin. I'm not talking about stevia and non-GMO erythritol or xylitol, I'm talking about aspartame and Splenda or worse. You can make your own sodas with other alternative sweeteners, using carbonated water and liquid flavored stevia.

What can I do about ketosis and constipation?

There are many scenarios that can cause constipation with the ketogenic diet. Most people assume it's a fiber issue. But it's not that simple. You want to compare what you were doing before ketosis and after. Look at the change in vegetable fiber consumption. If you don't have enough gut microbiomes to digest all these vegetables, it will cause bloating, constipation, gas, and all kinds of digestive issues.

Some people can do vegetables and others can't, of course. Some people can't do cabbage, others can't do cruciferous. So you might have to switch to less fibrous vegetables like various kinds of lettuce, especially kale and beet greens—for more potassium. Electrolytes greatly help with the constipation too. If you need more help with getting electrolytes, try my electrolyte powder. It helps you get that 4,700 mgs a day of potassium you need, which is hard to manage without a LOT of vegetable consumption.

What do I do about bad breath on a keto diet?

When you're burning more ketones, you can start releasing a bit of acetone, which smells like nail polish remover. Or you might release ammonia. Sometimes you get that sulfur smell. For all of these, increase vegetable consumption. Over time, you'll be more efficient at burning ketones, and a lot less of this will happen. If you're getting that ammonia smell, you're getting too much protein. Cut back. For that sulfur odor, that's a gut issue. You need to regulate your gut bacteria. You need to take a type of probiotic called effective microbiomes (EM). You can get it from the company called Teraganix.

What are the best supplements to take while on keto?

There are several healthy supplements that I recommend, most of them found on my website, drberg.com. These can help you avoid the side-effects that can develop when you start burning your own fat.

- Electrolyte Powder: this is loaded with electrolytes to provide your cells with the right nutrients

- Insulin and Glucose Support Formula: this supports healthy blood sugar levels to enhance the ketosis state.

- Nutritional Yeast: this has all the B vitamins you need and more.

- Wheat Grass Juice Powder: this is packed with vitamins and minerals as well as phytonutrients.

Can I chew gum?

This is a minor concern but yes.
You should choose (sorry, bad pun) xylitol gum.

Is lemon water okay?

Yes.

Can I have a cheat day?

No. If you want to get and stay in ketosis, you need to stick to the plan. It can take over a week to get back into ketosis after a sugar slip.

What do I do about a keto rash?

Typically, this is caused by the liver dumping something—the reason for that is you're losing lots of fat, and toxins are stored in your fat. As they come out of the system, these can cause a rash. The solution? Consume more vegetables. Also, try bentonite clay. This clay attracts toxins by pulling them toward itself, and excreted through the stool.

What kind of liquids should I be drinking that won't interfere with ketosis?

Filtered or spring water.

Bone broth is good—even in between fasting. Too much can slow ketosis for some people.

Homemade sodas with flavored xylitol—these are great. I have all kinds of videos on them.

Apple cider vinegar in water is great for helping you manage insulin and good for overcoming insulin resistance.

Unsweetened almond milk? Yes.

But avoid ALCOHOL and coconut water.

Can my cholesterol increase high on a ketogenic diet?

When you lose weight, fat cells shrink. In a fat cell, there are triglycerides and cholesterol. Now, as that fat cell shrinks, you can burn triglycerides, but you cannot burn cholesterol. So it will go into the blood, go to the liver, and come out through the bile. But you'll be totally fine, as long as your triglycerides are low—if you're not using those as fuel, then you're eating too much sugar. All that means is you're burning more fat! It will level out and come back to normal.

What about the bulletproof coffee?

Bulletproof coffee is coffee with added butter or coconut oil. If you want to use that as a meal, fine. But if you're trying to do IF or keto, anything can trigger insulin. That being said, I think it is good to do in the beginning as it reduces hunger, however for some people it could slow progress, so experiment.

What kind of cracker can I consume?

Finn Crisp Thin Rye Crispbread. It has got four net carbs, and in SMALL amounts, this is okay. You can find it online and at some stores.

What is ketoacidosis? Is this good or bad?

Ketoacidosis is a very dangerous condition that happens only when you're a type I diabetic and completely stop making insulin. This results is raising your acid levels far beyond normal. However, healthy ketosis will not produce acid levels even close to the condition ketoacidosis.

Can I eat beets, corn, tomatoes, and peas on a keto diet?

Try to limit beets, peas, and carrots. However, in small quantities, they are fine. Tomatoes are moderately sweeter and can be consumed in higher amounts than these others. But avoid potatoes and corn.

What mistakes are common with IF?

- Not eating enough vegetables!
- Not eating enough fat at the first meal of the day, to keep hunger and cravings away until your next meal.
- Thinking to yourself, "This is working so well that I can change it up, add foods, or tinker with the formula." In short, folks, if it ain't broke, don't fix it.

I'm losing weight but want to lose weight a bit faster with IF. How?

- Potassium; this is THE MOST IMPORTANT mineral to help you fix INSULIN and burn fat.
- Don't overeat. Don't gorge. Add more fat at meals to curb hunger.
- Get extra sleep; you burn fat during SLEEP. More sleep, and you wake up lighter.
- HIIT (high intense interval training, Tabata, sprints, etc.) burns fat

and majorly speeds the metabolism.

- Do it gradually, and be patient. Your body is trying to manufacture enzymes so you can run on fat. This can take six weeks for sugar junkies.

When should I exercise with IF?

With IF, the whole goal is to burn off excess fat, right? Watch how you feel when you exercise. Do you feel best after you eat or if you exercise while fasting? Watch if your legs feel heavy or if you tire too easily. Some people do well with eating first, and some love that feeling of exercising fasted and eating afterward.

Can I do IF without doing a keto diet—or should I do both?

Well, if you're doing IF alone, but you're eating lots of carbohydrates and not eating nutrient-dense foods, your skin, hair, and nails will suffer. Plus, you have to deal with the toxic effect of certain foods.

Can I get hypoglycemia (low blood sugar) from IF?

IF actually improves hypoglycemia and high blood sugar problems!

Will IF mess up my thyroid?

No, but going low calorie will. As long as you're having very nutrient-dense meals twice a day, your body will be fine. What your thyroid does not like is starvation mode. Starvation just signals the body to slow the metabolism.

HELP! I'm way too hungry!

Hunger is one way to know if you're in fat burning, because the longer you do keto, the less hungry you'll be. If you're getting severe hunger with weakness and brain fog, you're not quite into keto. Back off a bit. Don't be doing 20-hour fasts. You need more fuel to give your body the energy it needs to even manufacture the ENZYMES to burn FAT instead of glucose. Take it slow, add more fat to your first meal, and eat nutrient-dense foods. If you need more nutrients—try adding some nutritional yeast AND electrolytes and major amounts of potassium, which will help you fix insulin resistance and help you get into fat burning. Bone broth is great for a snack. It's nutrients without calories, period.

What boosts more growth hormone (GH), IF or high intensity interval training (HIIT)?

Although they are both very effective at stimulating an anabolic hormone release that burns fat and builds lean muscle, IF actually is superior, releasing 350–2,000% more GH than exercise of any kind.

What about the gallbladder—is IF good or bad for the gallbladder?

IF is very good for the gallbladder in all kinds of ways. Gallstones are caused by two things: high insulin and low bile. IF both lowers insulin spikes and concentrates bile to make it easier to digest fats and absorb nutrients from the foods you eat. If you're eating five times a day, you're using up your bile reserves like crazy.

Can I do a keto diet and IF without a gallbladder?

Some people actually grow a gallbladder back! Really! But in general, IF combined with ketosis actually helps the gallbladder. However, when you only do ketosis, you have the combination of higher fats but not IF, and the frequent eating can add additional stress on the gallbladder.

Thanks for reading, and all the best of luck with your new lifestyle!!

Dr. Berg